Managing Chronic Pain

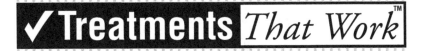

Managing Chronic Pain

A Cognitive-Behavioral Therapy Approach

Workbook

John D. Otis

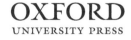

UNIVERSITY PRESS

2007

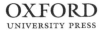

OXFORD
UNIVERSITY PRESS

Oxford University Press, Inc., publishes works that further
Oxford University's objective of excellence
in research, scholarship, and education.

Oxford   New York
Auckland   Cape Town   Dar es Salaam   Hong Kong   Karachi
Kuala Lumpur   Madrid   Melbourne   Mexico City   Nairobi
New Delhi   Shanghai   Taipei   Toronto

With offices in
Argentina   Austria   Brazil   Chile   Czech Republic   France   Greece
Guatemala   Hungary   Italy   Japan   Poland   Portugal   Singapore
South Korea   Switzerland   Thailand   Turkey   Ukraine   Vietnam

Copyright © 2007 by Oxford University Press, Inc.

Published by Oxford University Press, Inc.
198 Madison Avenue, New York, New York 10016

www.oup.com

Oxford is a registered trademark of Oxford University Press

ISBN 978-0-19-532917-9

19 18 17 16 15 14 13 12 11

Printed in the United States of America
on acid-free paper

About Treatments*ThatWork*™

One of the most difficult problems confronting patients with various disorders and diseases is finding the best help available. Everyone is aware of friends or family who have sought treatment from a seemingly reputable practitioner, only to find out later from another doctor that the original diagnosis was wrong or the treatments recommended were inappropriate or perhaps even harmful. Most patients, or family members, address this problem by reading everything they can about their symptoms, seeking information on the Internet, or aggressively "asking around" to tap knowledge from friends and acquaintances. Governments and healthcare policymakers are also aware that people in need don't always get the best treatments, something they refer to as "variability in healthcare practices."

Now healthcare systems around the world are attempting to correct this variability by introducing "evidence-based practice." This simply means that it is in everyone's interest that patients get the most up-to-date and effective care for a particular problem. Healthcare policymakers have also recognized that it is very useful to give consumers of healthcare as much information as possible so that they can make intelligent decisions in a collaborative effort to improve health and mental health. This series, Treatments *ThatWork*™, is designed to accomplish just that. Only the latest and most effective interventions for particular problems are described, in user-friendly language. To be included in this series, each treatment program must pass the highest standards of evidence available, as determined by a scientific advisory board. Thus, when individuals suffering from these problems or their family members seek out an expert clinician who is familiar with these interventions and decides that they are appropriate, they will have confidence that they are receiving the best care available. Of course, only your healthcare professional can decide on the right mix of treatments for you.

This program presents a cognitive-behavioral therapy (CBT) approach to chronic pain management. Medical treatment is often not enough to relieve the very real physical and emotional suffering associated with chronic pain. Each session of this program teaches a new skill you can use to help manage chronic pain that will complement your medical treatment. With practice, these techniques can help reduce your pain and increase your ability to cope. This program helps you take control of your pain, which can improve the quality of your life as well as decrease your reliance on medical interventions. This program is most effective when carried out in collaboration with your clinician.

David H. Barlow, Editor-in-Chief
Treatments *ThatWork*™
Boston, Massachusetts

Contents

Chapter 1   *Overview of the Program*

Goals

- To learn about the program
- To understand what the program will involve
- To determine if this program is right for you

Purpose of this Program

Pain is usually temporary; however, for some people pain persists over time and is considered chronic. Chronic pain can create a reliance on medication and cause emotional distress. It can also affect a person's ability to engage in occupational, social, or recreational activities. A lack of activity can contribute to increased isolation, depression, and physical deconditioning, all of which can make the experience of pain even worse. This program is designed not only to help you reduce pain, but also to increase your activity level and improve your overall quality of life.

Cognitive-Behavioral Therapy

This program uses a cognitive-behavioral therapy (CBT) approach that has been proven effective for the management of chronic pain. CBT for pain management takes an active problem-solving approach to tackling the many challenges associated with the experience of chronic pain. Rather than seeing yourself as helpless and disabled because of your pain, CBT encourages you to take back control and re-engage in activities. There are several key components to CBT for chronic pain, including:

- Cognitive restructuring (learning how to recognize cognitive errors and change unhelpful negative thoughts related to pain into more positive coping thoughts)

- Relaxation training (e.g., breathing, visual imagery, progressive muscle relaxation)

- Time-based activity pacing (learning how to become more active without overdoing it)

- Homework assignments designed to decrease avoidance of activity and reintroduce a healthier, more active lifestyle

The Role of Medications

One of the goals of this program is to teach you skills so that you can manage pain on your own; however, you do not have to stop taking your medication to participate in this program. You may find that as you learn ways to manage pain on your own, you are able to reduce your reliance on pain medication. If you would like to change your medication during this program, you should discuss this first with your physician.

Outline of This Program

This program is divided into 11 sessions, each teaching a new skill for coping with chronic pain. Each chapter of this workbook corresponds to a particular session and includes information and instructions for mastering skills. Homework exercises will help you apply the skills learned in session. The workbook includes all worksheets and monitoring forms used during the program. All forms intended for multiple use can be photocopied from the workbook or downloaded from the Treatments *ThatWork*™ Web site at www.oup.com/us/ttw.

You will also be setting personal goals that you would like to achieve during the program. You will be taking small steps toward these goals each week until they are reached. In order for this program to be effective, you will need to make a commitment to making the time and effort to learn new skills and work toward your goals.

Is this Program Right for You?

Before beginning this program, your therapist will ask you to complete some assessment measures. These questionnaires will ask you about the history of your pain, the impact pain has on your life, your efforts to cope with pain, and other factors that may affect your pain experience. The assessment will help your therapist understand your pain condition and determine if you could benefit from therapy.

Chronic pain can be the result of a physical injury or associated with diseases like cancer. It can also be part of neuropathic conditions that involve damage to nerves that carry information about pain. Chronic pain can occur in many parts of the body, and each pain condition has its own characteristics. Low back pain, knee pain, tension headaches, and migraine headaches are common chronic pain complaints. No matter what the cause or type of condition, however, this program can help you learn how to effectively manage chronic pain.

Chapter 2

Session 1: Education on Chronic Pain

Goals

- To review assessment results
- To discuss the impact pain has on your life
- To understand the pain cycle
- To set goals for treatment

Overview

The session will begin with a review of your pretreatment assessment results. Next you will discuss the different ways pain affects your life. You will also learn about how thoughts, feelings, and behaviors maintain the cycle of pain. Last, with the help of your therapist, you will set goals for treatment.

Assessment Review

At the start of the session, your therapist will review with you the results of the assessment measures you completed before beginning therapy. You and the therapist will discuss your strengths in coping with pain and areas where you could improve your skills.

The Impact of Pain

It is important to note that pain can be experienced both physically and emotionally. People with chronic pain, or pain that persists for three months or longer, often find that pain affects more than just their neck, shoulder, or back. It can affect everything they do—the way they work, the way they play, the way they think, and the way they feel. You may have noticed this in your own life.

The effects of pain generally fall under the broad categories of *activities* and *thoughts and feelings:*

Activities: Pain can affect a person's activity level and the types of work or social activities a person performs, and this can have an impact on a person's experience of pain. For example, a person in pain may avoid socializing with others, call in sick to work, have a hard time getting out of bed, watch TV all day, and so forth. This can lead to decreased muscle tone, weight gain, and overall weakness. Questions you might want to think about include:

- Has pain affected your ability to engage in social activities or hobbies?
- Has pain affected your ability to work or function?
- When in pain, what kinds of activities do you usually do?
- Has limiting your activities resulted in any negative physical or social effects?

Thoughts and Feelings: The way a person thinks (e.g., "Life is unfair," "I'm never going to get better") and feels (e.g., worthless, depressed, anxious) can have a big impact on his experience of pain. Research indicates that negative emotions or thoughts tend to increase the focus on pain so that it is more noticeable. Consider the following questions:

- Have you ever observed a relationship between your emotions and pain?
- How do you feel emotionally on days when you are experiencing a lot of pain?
- Does anger, frustration, or sadness also increase with the pain?
- What kinds of thoughts are associated with those feelings?

Complete the Things that Affect My Pain worksheet to help increase your awareness of how activities, thoughts, feelings, or other events can affect your experience of pain. Notice if any of these things are under your control.

Things that Affect My Pain

Your assignment for this session is to make a list of all the things you can think of that you believe affect your pain. Can you think of things that make your pain decrease? How about things that make your pain increase? These can be things you did or thoughts you had during the day. Please write down these things in the spaces below.

Things that can make my pain INCREASE:

Doing too much   worry getting frustrated   Worrying about a relationship   Too much exercise at gym   To much work at home

Things that can make my pain DECREASE:

relax - laying down an hour   a Tylenol

The Cycle of Pain, Distress and Disability

The pain cycle shown in Figure 2.1 demonstrates the relationship between pain, distress (thoughts and feelings), and disability (behaviors).

When pain persists over time, you may develop negative beliefs about your pain (e.g., "This is never going to get better," "I can't cope with my pain") or negative thoughts about yourself (e.g., "I'm worthless to my family because I can't work," "I'm never going to recover"). As pain continues, you may avoid doing activities (e.g., work, social activities, or hobbies) for fear of further injury or increases in pain. As you withdraw and become less active, your muscles may become weaker, you may begin to gain or lose weight, and your overall physical conditioning may decline. The pain cycle diagram shows how distress and disability feed back into pain and make it seem worse.

General Goals of Treatment

The general goals of this treatment program are:

- To reduce the impact pain has on your daily life

- To learn skills for coping better with pain

- To improve your physical and emotional functioning

- To reduce your pain and reliance on pain medication

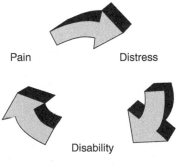

Figure 2.1
Pain Cycle

This program will teach you many techniques in order to achieve these goals. We have seen that your thoughts and activities play an important part in your experience of pain. It is important to recognize that your thoughts and the things you do in response to pain are all under your control. By learning ways of addressing negative thoughts and emotions associated with pain, and ways of keeping active, you will gain greater control over your pain and your life.

Remember, in order to effectively learn new techniques, it is important to practice both in session and at home. Completing the homework will help you get the most out of the program.

Setting Your Personal Overall Goals for Treatment

Besides the general goals of this program, you will want to set your own overall behavioral goals for therapy. These should be goals that you can reasonably achieve over the course of therapy and can be any positive behavior that you would like to increase. For example, they can be something you have done in the past but would like to do more often, something you have been meaning to do but have been putting off, or something you have never done but would like to try. You may also want to set a goal in one of the areas you need to work on according to the assessment results. Keep in mind that it is important to set specific, rather than vague, goals (e.g., "walk one mile every day" vs. "be a better person"). Use the Goal Setting Worksheet found in this chapter to record your goals. You may photocopy this form from the book or download multiple copies from the Treatments *ThatWork*™ Web site at www.oup.com/us/ttw. Identify what you would consider some improvement, moderate improvement, and maximum improvement toward each goal.

Your therapist will help you break down your overall treatment goals into weekly behavioral goals. These small, achievable goals will help you work step by step toward the overall goals. For example, if one of your overall treatment goals is to walk a mile, a weekly behavioral goal might be to buy a good pair of walking sneakers and walk a quarter of a mile two mornings that week. The next week's goal

Goal Setting Worksheet

Goal	Some Improvement	Moderate Improvement	Maximum Improvement
1.			
2.			
3.			
4.			
5.			

might then be to walk a half-mile three mornings that week. Record your weekly behavioral goals in the space provided in the homework section.

Homework

✎ Complete the Things that Affect My Pain worksheet.

✎ Work toward completing the weekly behavioral goals set at the end of the session.

Travel again
more meditation
Be sure + make gym 3x a wk
Knee Surgery

Behavioral Goals for the Week
1.
2.
3.
4.
5.

Chapter 3

Session 2: Theories of Pain and Diaphragmatic Breathing

Goals

■ To learn about theories of pain

■ To practice diaphragmatic breathing

Overview

To begin, your therapist will review your homework from the past week, including your weekly goals and completed Things that Affect My Pain worksheet. In the first part of this session, your therapist will introduce you to theories of pain. The rest of the session will be spent learning and practicing diaphragmatic breathing.

Theories of Pain

To understand your pain, it is helpful to know about current theories of pain. Our discussion centers around two theories of pain: the specificity theory and the gate control theory.

Specificity Theory

The specificity theory suggests that the amount of pain a person feels is directly related to the amount of tissue damage that has occurred. According to this theory, pain should stop when the tissue has healed. However, there are several problems with this theory:

1. Many people continue to feel pain after injuries have healed. For example, patients who undergo the amputation of a limb may experience phantom pain or discomfort seemingly caused by the missing limb. If there is a direct relationship between pain and tissue damage, this should not happen.

2. People with similar amounts of tissue damage experience different levels of pain. This suggests that there is something unique about every person that affects the amount of pain experienced.

3. Some people with very little tissue damage feel a great deal of pain, while others with considerable tissue damage feel no pain.

The Gate Control Theory

The gate control theory was developed in the early 1960s by Ronald Melzack and Patrick Wall to account for the importance of the mind and brain in pain perception (see Figure 3.1). When you are injured a signal travels from the site of injury through nerve fibers to the spinal cord, and then up to the brain. The brain interprets the signal about tissue damage and you perceive pain. The gate control theory

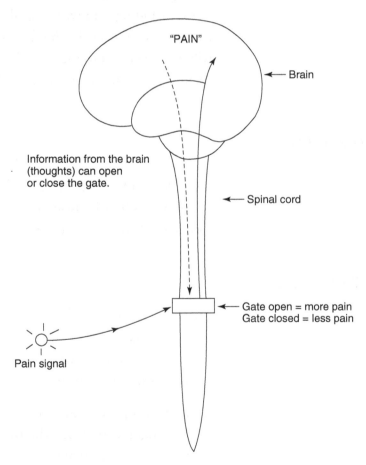

Figure 3.1

The Gate Control Theory

Table 3.1 Things that Open the Gate

Physical	Degenerative changes, muscle tension, drug abuse
Cognitive	Attention to pain, thoughts about uncontrollability of pain, beliefs about pain as a mysterious, terrible thing
Emotions	Depression, fear/anxiety, anger
Activity	Too much or too little activity, poor diet and other health behaviors, imbalance between work, social, and recreational activity
Social	Little support from family and friends, others focusing on your pain, others trying to protect you too much

suggests that there is a type of "gate" in the spinal cord that can open and close based on input from the brain and the body. The opening and closing of the gate modifies how much information is sent to the brain from an injured area. Negative thoughts open the gate, which lets more pain information through, while positive thoughts close the gate and restrict the pain message. The result is that pain signals can be intensified, reduced, or even blocked on their way to the brain.

[handwritten margin note: Neg positive]

Note that attention to pain tends to hold the gate open, so when you are bored or unoccupied, you may notice an increase in pain. On the other hand, when you are distracted or busy with an enjoyable activity, you may not experience as much pain. That's because information from the brain is competing with information from the injury and closing the gate. Sensory information can also close the gate. This is why when you bump your shin, rubbing it often helps. When you rub your knee you are stimulating different types of nerves at the

Table 3.2 Things that Close the Gate

Physical	Drugs, surgery, reduced muscular tension
Cognitive	Distraction or external focus of attention, thoughts of control over pain, beliefs about pain as predictable and manageable
Emotions	Emotional stability, relaxation, and calm, positive mood
Activity	Appropriate pacing of activity, positive health habits, balance between work, recreation, rest, and social activity
Social	Support from others, reasonable involvement from family and friends, encouragement from others to maintain moderate activity

site of injury. These nerves send a signal to close the gate so less pain information can get through to the brain. See tables 3.1 and 3.2 for a more complete list of things that open and close the pain gate.

Diaphragmatic Breathing

This program will introduce you to several relaxation techniques that can help you gain more control over your body. The health benefits of relaxation include increased energy, decreased muscle tension and fatigue, improved sleep, lower blood pressure, and decreased pain. People often think that learning to relax means that you have to slow down or be less productive, but in fact if you are relaxed you can think more clearly and function better.

Learning to breathe correctly is probably the easiest and most effective method of learning how to relax. Although breathing is automatic, as people get older they sometimes develop the habit of taking short, shallow breaths. This often results from increased muscle tension in times of stress or pain. This type of breathing delivers less oxygen to your body and can cause your chest and shoulder muscles to work even harder. However, you can train yourself to breathe in a way that helps you relax and reduce your pain.

A different way of breathing is "diaphragmatic breathing," which requires you to use the muscles in your diaphragm and abdomen. The diaphragm is a dome-shaped muscle located right under your rib cage, between your chest cavity and stomach cavity. During correct diaphragmatic breathing the diaphragm is tightened and pulls the lower part of your lungs down so that more air can be inhaled. As you inhale, the abdomen swells (your stomach is pushed out a little), the rib cage expands, and at the end of the inhalation the upper chest expands. If you ever watch babies or small children sleep, you will notice that it is their bellies, not their chests, that rise and fall as they breathe.

Steps to Diaphragmatic Breathing

1. *Set up a relaxation area*: First, find a quiet place where you will not be disturbed. If needed, take the phone off the hook and tell others to give you this time alone. Loosen any tight

clothing, or change into comfortable clothes. Next, sit with your feet flat on the floor and your hands in your lap or on the arms of the chair. You don't want to lie down because you might fall asleep, and learning can occur only if you are awake. Make sure you start out in a comfortable position.

2. *Monitor*: Place one hand on your abdomen and one hand on your chest. Take a normal breath in and notice which hand moves the most. Most likely it will be the hand on your chest, and this indicates that you tend to breathe shallow breaths from your chest as mentioned. Now try to take a breath from your abdomen—you might feel as though you are pushing your stomach out, and that is the way it should feel.

Alternatively you can place both of your hands across your abdomen so that the tips of the middle fingers are just touching near the center of the stomach. If you are breathing correctly, the tips of the fingers should separate.

3. *Practice*: Now close your eyes if you are comfortable doing so. Take a deep breath in through your nose slowly for a count of three and then exhale for a count of three from your mouth. Your exhalation should be as long in duration as your inhalation. Continue breathing in a comfortable pace, remembering to breathe in through the nose for a count of three and out through the mouth for a count of three. If you begin to feel dizzy, try breathing less deeply and at a more normal rate.

You may want to repeat some of the following statements to yourself to help you relax while breathing:

■ With each breath I feel my body sinking into the chair.

■ With each breath I scan my body for places of tension and let those areas relax.

■ With each breath my body feels heavier and warmer.

■ With each breath I feel myself becoming more relaxed and calm.

■ I can feel relaxed like this whenever I want, just by taking the time to breathe deeply.

Try using this technique at a consistent time and place where you will not be disturbed (e.g., every morning before breakfast while sitting in the easy chair, sitting on the deck outside before the kids come home from school). Once you have practiced sufficiently and learned to use the breathing to become relaxed, you can start using the technique at other times during the day. In this way, you will get used to using the technique on a regular basis and in different situations. In addition, after continued practice you will require less time to become relaxed.

You may have already tried to use breathing at a time when you were really "stressed out" but it didn't work. This is probably because you hadn't learned to use breathing to relax first. Give yourself a chance to really practice before expecting breathing to be very effective when up against very strong emotions. Remember, you have had years to learn how to be stressed, but only a little practice at relaxation.

Homework

✎ Practice diaphragmatic breathing using the Breathing Practice Log.

✎ Work toward completing the weekly behavioral goals set at the end of the session.

Behaviorial Goals for the Week
1. _____
2. _____
3. _____
4. _____
5. _____

Breathing Practice Log

The assignment for this week is to:

1. Practice your breathing exercise _____ times, for _____ minutes.

2. Rate your relaxation level before and after, using the rating scale below.

3. Record the total time spent relaxing.

Rating Scale

0 ——————————————————— 10

Not at all relaxed   Completely relaxed

Date	Relaxation Rating Before	Relaxation Rating After	Total Time Practicing
1/2/07	4	9	13 min

Chapter 4　　　　*Session 3: Progressive Muscle*
Relaxation and Visual Imagery

Goals

- To learn progressive muscle relaxation (PMR)
- To practice visual imagery

Overview

This session introduces two relaxation techniques. In the first half of the session, you will learn progressive muscle relaxation (PMR). The rest of the session will be spent doing a visual imagery exercise.

Progressive Muscle Relaxation (PMR)

The most common response to an acute painful injury is to tighten the muscles. The tightening acts to limit movement, protect the body, and allow time for healing. However, when pain is chronic, this response can cause problems by increasing muscle tension over the long run. Anger, anxiety, frustration, and stress can also increase muscle tension. Increased muscle tension can make chronic pain worse, as well as lead to feeling fatigued and impatient.

Common places to hold tension include the neck, shoulders, and back; however, most of us are not aware of when these muscles are tense. The purpose of progressive muscle relaxation (PMR) is to help you to develop an awareness of when your muscles are becoming tense and learn to relax them before the tension becomes great. PMR involves going through groups of muscles in turn, tensing them for a few seconds, and very gradually releasing the tension. This technique not only decreases muscle tension, but also induces a general state of mental calm and deep physical relaxation.

You may find that the basic procedure takes a few attempts to get used to, but once it is mastered you will be able to relax your muscles rapidly. Instead of performing PMR on individual muscles (e.g., hand, forearm, and biceps), you may be able to tense an entire muscle group like an arm or leg and achieve the same result.

Use the following instructions, along with the Progressive Muscle Relaxation Practice Log provided at the end of the chapter, to practice at home. You may photocopy this log from the book or download multiple copies from the Treatments *That Work*™ Web site at www.oup.com/us/ttw. If you feel pain in specific areas after this exercise, do not tense that muscle group, or perform only mild tensing in that area the next time.

How to Begin

Make yourself as comfortable as possible in a seated position. Sit up straight with good posture, hands resting in your lap. Start with diaphragmatic breathing, inhaling and exhaling deeply. When you are ready, begin tensing and relaxing specific muscle groups. For feet, legs, arms, and hands, tense one side at a time. If you are right-handed, start with your right side. If you are left-handed, start with your left side.

Relaxation of the Feet

1. Flex your foot by pulling your toes up toward your knees while your feet are on the floor.

2. Feel the tension building in your foot and hold it for three seconds.

3. Take a deep breath.

4. As you exhale, say the word "relax" and release the tension slowly, paying close attention to the different sensations.

Perform this twice and repeat with the other foot.

Relaxation of the Calves

1. Contract the calf muscle by lifting the heel of your foot.

2. Feel the tension build and hold it for three seconds.

3. Take a deep breath.

4. As you exhale, say the word "relax" and release the tension gradually by letting your heel return to the floor. Notice the different sensations.

Perform this twice and repeat with the other calf muscle.

Relaxation of the Knees and Upper Thighs

1. Extend your leg out straight and tense your thigh muscle.

2. Feel the tension building in your thigh and hold it for three seconds.

3. Take a deep breath.

4. As you exhale, say the word "relax" and release the tension, lowering your leg to the floor.

Perform this twice and repeat with the other thigh.

Relaxation of the Abdomen

1. Observe your abdomen rising and falling with each breath.

2. Inhale deeply and tense the abdomen (stomach muscles).

3. Feel the tension and hold it for three seconds.

4. As you exhale, say the word "relax" and release the tension in your abdomen.

Relaxation of the Hands

1. Tightly clench your fist for about five seconds.

2. Focus on the sensations in your hand and examine the feelings of muscular tension.

3. Take a deep breath, and as you exhale release the tension slowly and gradually, allowing your fist to open and your fingers to move.

4. Take a few moments to allow feelings of relaxation to develop. Focus on the contrast between relaxation and tension.

Perform this twice and repeat using the other hand.

Relaxation of the Forearms

1. Turn your palm face up, make a tight fist, and curl it toward you.

2. Feel the tension build and hold it for three seconds.

3. Take a deep breath.

4. As you exhale, say the word "relax" and release the tension in your forearm and hand.

Perform this twice and repeat with the other forearm.

Relaxation of the Biceps

1. Bring your fist in toward your shoulder and tighten your bicep.

2. Feel the tension build and hold it for three seconds.

3. Take a deep breath.

4. As you exhale, say the word "relax" and release the tension in your bicep while also relaxing your forearm and unclenching your fist. Let your entire arm go completely relaxed.

Perform this twice and repeat with the other bicep.

Relaxation of the Shoulders

1. Draw the shoulder blades together (to midline of body).

2. Contract the muscles across the upper back.

3. Feel the tension build and hold it for three seconds.

4. Take a deep breath.

5. As you exhale, say the word "relax" and release the tension, letting the shoulder blades return to their normal position, almost as if a weight had been placed on them.

Relaxation of the Jaw and Facial Muscles

1. Clench your teeth together.

2. Tense the muscles in the back of your jaw.

3. Turn the corners of your mouth into a tight smile.

4. Wrinkle the bridge of your nose and squeeze your eyes shut.

5. Tense all facial muscles in toward the center of your face.

6. Take a deep breath.

7. As you exhale, say the word "relax" and release the tension in your jaw and face.

Relaxation of the Forehead

1. Raise your eyebrows up and tense the muscles across the forehead and scalp.

2. Feel the tension build and hold it for three seconds.

3. Take a deep breath.

4. As you exhale, say the word "relax" and release the tension.

Whole Body Muscle Relaxation

1. Focus on relaxation flowing from the top of your head:

2. Over your face

3. Down the back of your neck and shoulders

4. Over your chest and abdomen

5. Flowing through your arms and hands

6. Flowing through your hips and buttocks

7. Into your thighs, knees, and calves

8. Into your ankles and feet.

9. Continue to deep breathe quietly for a few minutes.

Finishing the PMR Exercise

Take a few seconds to empty your mind and to allow the feelings of relaxation to spread throughout your body. Scan your body, and if you find any remaining tension allow yourself to let go of it. Count backwards in your head from three to one:

3. Become aware of your surroundings.

2. Move your feet, legs, hands, and arms. Rotate your head.

1. Open your eyes slowly, feeling refreshed and relaxed.

Visual Imagery

Stress and tension can be reduced significantly by using your imagination and focusing on positive, healing images. The purpose of this technique is to help you create a relaxing image that you can think of on your own. The image can be any scene you like, but it must be a pleasant image that you can visualize. For example, some people like to imagine a beach scene, while others prefer to imagine being in the woods, vacationing with friends, or being in a warm kitchen with cookies baking in the oven. This technique requires practice and good concentration in order for the visual image to be effective. Use the Imagery Form to help you imagine the scene.

In session, the therapist will guide you in imagining your chosen scene. When practicing visual imagery at home, use the following instructions along with the Visual Imagery Practice Log provided at the end of the chapter. You may photocopy this form from the book or download multiple copies from the Treatments *That Work*™ Web site at www.oup.com/us/ttw.

Prepare

Make yourself as comfortable as possible in your chair. Shift your focus to the image you have chosen. To begin, take several deep breaths.

Describe the Image

As you visualize the scene, notice what you hear, smell, and taste. Imagine that you are reaching out and touching the things around you. Identify a path along which you travel through your place. Move deeper and deeper into the image. Feel the calm and peacefulness of the scene. Notice how your body feels, so you can return to this feeling next time.

Imagery Form

Record information about the image in the spaces provided. Include specific details in order to help create the scene.

Place: *Where do you want to be? (e.g., beach, forest)*

_____

Vision: *What do you see? (e.g., trees, grass, sun, people, animals)*

_____

_____

Smell: *What do you smell? (e.g., ocean, pine, flowers)*

_____

_____

Sounds: *What do you hear? (e.g., birds, sticks cracking, waves)*

_____

_____

Touch: *What do you feel? (e.g., cool breeze, warm sun, water)*

_____

_____

Taste: *What can you taste? (e.g., salty air, sweet berries, cool water)*

_____

_____

Other:

_____

_____

_____

_____

_____

Finish the Exercise

Take a few seconds to empty your mind and to allow the feelings of relaxation to spread throughout your body. Scan your body, and if you find any remaining tension allow yourself to let go of it. Count backwards in your head from three to one as you become more alert. Open your eyes slowly, feeling refreshed and relaxed.

Homework

✎ Practice PMR using the Progressive Muscle Relaxation Practice Log.

✎ Practice imagery using the Visual Imagery Practice Log.

✎ Work toward completing the weekly behavioral goals set at the end of the session.

Behavioral Goals for the Week

1. _____

2. _____

3. _____

4. _____

5. _____

Progressive Muscle Relaxation Practice Log

The assignment for this week is to:

1. Practice PMR _____ times, for _____ minutes.

2. Rate your relaxation level before and after, using the rating scale below.

3. Record the total time spent practicing.

Rating Scale

0 —————————————————————————— 10

Not at all relaxed   Completely relaxed

Date	Relaxation Rating Before	Relaxation Rating After	Total Time Practicing
1/3/07	2	7	15 min

Muscle Groups:

Feet	Abdomen	Shoulders
Calves	Hands	Jaw and face
Thighs	Forearms	Forehead
	Biceps	Whole body

Visual Imagery Practice Log

The assignment for this week is to:

1. Practice imagery _____ times, for _____ minutes.

2. Rate your relaxation level before and after, using the rating scale below.

3. Record the total time spent practicing.

Rating Scale

0 ——————————————————————— 10

Not at all relaxed   Completely relaxed

Date	Relaxation Rating Before	Relaxation Rating After	Total Time Practicing
1/4/07	3	8	10 min

Chapter 5

Session 4: Automatic Thoughts and Pain

Goals

- To learn about automatic thoughts
- To understand the relationship between thoughts, emotions, and pain
- To identify cognitive errors
- To practice using the ABC model

Overview

This session introduces the concept of automatic thoughts. You will learn how to identify common errors in your thinking. You will then use the ABC model to examine the relationship between events, beliefs, and consequences.

Automatic Thoughts

Automatic thoughts are thoughts that we have immediately after getting any kind of information. They occur very quickly, and unless we make an effort to pay attention to them, we may not even be aware of them. We have automatic thoughts for everything that goes on in our world, even for very trivial kinds of things. For example, suppose one afternoon you arrange to meet a friend back at your place to have lunch. You go home and as you get closer to your door, you see that there's a piece of paper taped to it. The kinds of automatic thoughts that you have are affected by the kinds of experiences you've had. So, for instance, if you have a lot of friends who let you down, you might be more apt to have an automatic thought that the note was from your friend canceling lunch, rather than a note from

UPS or a neighbor. In this way, automatic thoughts help us to make sense of the world.

Thoughts, Emotions, and Pain

Though automatic thoughts have a purpose, they can sometimes be negative and based on faulty information. They can trigger even more negative thoughts that can have an impact on how we feel and how we behave. You may think someone *makes* you mad, but it's what you *think* about that person's actions that causes you to feel angry. You might even find out later that the reason for your anger turned out not to be true. The way you think about an event, either positively or negatively, determines the emotions you experience. Negative thoughts lead to negative emotions, while pleasant emotions are caused by thinking pleasant thoughts. Figure 5.1 shows the chain of events.

As we discussed in Session 2 with the gate control theory, thoughts and emotions can have an impact on pain. Negative thoughts/emotions cause the gate to open so that more pain information gets to the brain, while positive thoughts/emotions cause the gate to close and result in less pain. You may have noticed a relationship between your emotions and your pain. For example, when you're angry or frustrated pain seems to get worse, but when you're happy or busy enjoying yourself you feel less pain or don't even notice pain.

Cognitive Errors

We have learned that emotions can affect pain, and emotions are caused by how we think. The problem is that our automatic thoughts may be unreliable, causing us to experience negative emotions and pain

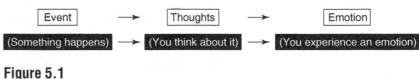

Figure 5.1
Chain of Events

unnecessarily. One way that we can manage pain, then, is to learn to identify inaccurate and negative thoughts that contribute to negative emotions and increased pain.

Cognitive errors are ways of thinking that are based on faulty assumptions or misconceptions. Making these types of errors is very common, and as you review the list some of these will probably seem very familiar. Note the ones that you think may apply to you.

List of Cognitive Errors (Adapted from Burns, 1999)

1. *All-or-nothing thinking:* When you see things in all-or-nothing categories. For example, if your performance falls short of perfect, you see yourself as a total failure.

2. *Overgeneralization:* When you see a single negative event as a never-ending pattern. For example, if you do not do well at one thing, you think you are not good at anything.

3. *Mental filter:* When you pick out a single negative detail and dwell on it exclusively, so that your vision of all reality becomes darkened. A good metaphor is a drop of ink that discolors the entire glass of water.

4. *Disqualifying the positive:* When you reject positive experiences by insisting they "don't count" for some reason or another. In this way, you can maintain a negative belief that is contradicted by your everyday experiences.

5. *Jumping to conclusions:* When you make a negative interpretation of an event even though there are no definite facts that convincingly support your conclusion.

    a. *Mind reading:* When you arbitrarily conclude that people are reacting negatively to you, and you do not bother to consider other possible explanations for their behavior (e.g., they are tired, they had a rough day).
    b. *The fortune-teller error:* When you anticipate that things will turn out badly, and you feel convinced that your prediction is an already established fact. This prediction may in turn affect your behavior, making it a self-fulfilling prophecy.

6. *Binocular vision:* When you distort information in such a way that you can no longer view the situation realistically.

   a. *Magnification:* When you exaggerate the importance of things (such as your goof-up, or someone else's achievement).

   b. *Minimization:* When you inappropriately shrink things (such as your own positive qualities or someone else's imperfections) until they appear tiny.

7. *Catastrophizing:* When you predict extreme and horrible consequences to the outcomes of events. For example, a turndown for a date means a life of utter isolation, or making a mistake at work means you will be fired for incompetence and never get another job.

8. *Emotional reasoning:* When you assume that your negative emotions necessarily reflect the way things really are. You might think, "I feel it; therefore, it must be true."

9. *"Should" statements:* When you try to motivate yourself with "shoulds" and "shouldn'ts." "Musts" and "oughts" are also offenders. The emotional consequence of this type of statement is guilt. When you direct "should" statements toward others, you feel anger, frustration, and resentment.

10. *Labeling and mislabeling:* This is an extreme form of overgeneralization. Instead of describing your error, you attach a negative label to yourself: "I'm a failure," "I'm stupid." When someone else's behavior rubs you the wrong way, you attach a negative label to him: "He's an idiot." Mislabeling involves describing an event with language that is highly colored and emotionally loaded: "That was a total disaster," "This has ruined my life."

11. *Personalization:* When you see negative events as indicative of some negative characteristic of yourself, or you see yourself as the cause of some negative external event for which, in fact, you were not primarily responsible: "I should have caught the error in the report before it left my boss's desk," "I'm bad luck; my team loses every time I watch the game."

12. *Maladaptive thoughts:* When you focus on something that may in fact be true, but is nonetheless not helpful to focus on exces-

sively: "My knee hasn't been the same since surgery," "I'm starting to lose my hair."

The ABC Model

Now that you know about cognitive errors, you probably want to learn how to stop making them. First you must practice making the connection between the way you think about an event and the way it makes you feel and act. This can be accomplished by using an ABC Worksheet, which has three columns:

- **A** is for Activating Event: This is the stressful situation that is happening.

- **B** is for Beliefs: These are things you tell yourself. They are the thoughts you have about the situation.

- **C** is for Consequences: These are the feelings and reactions you have in response to the Activating Event. These reactions can be emotional, physical, or behavioral, or all three.

You may photocopy this form from the workbook or download multiple copies from the Treatments *ThatWork*™ Web site at www.oup.com/us/ttw. Completing the ABC Worksheet will help you to become more aware of the consequences of negative thoughts. You will begin to see that negative thoughts make your experience of pain worse. In the next session, you will learn to replace these negative thoughts with more positive and healthy thoughts. This will help reduce negative emotions and can result in decreased pain.

Homework

✎ Use the ABC Worksheet to identify the beliefs and consequences associated with three activating events this week. At least one of the events must be related to pain.

✎ Work toward completing the weekly behavioral goals set at the end of the session.

List of cognitive errors adapted from Burns, D.D. (1999). *The Feeling Good Handbook.* (Rev. ed.) New York: Plume/Penguin Books.

Behavioral Goals for the Week

1. _____

2. _____

3. _____

4. _____

5. _____

ABC Worksheet

Activating Event (Stressful Situation)	Beliefs (Automatic Thoughts)	C (M
I bend over to pick up a package and I get a big increase in my pain.	Why me? What did I do to deserve this? Now I'm in for a miserable day.	**Emotional:** Frustrated **Physical:** Face feels hot and flushed **Behavioral:** Walk slowly so I don't cause more pain
		Emotional: **Physical:** **Behavioral:**
		Emotional: **Physical:** **Behavioral:**
		Emotional: **Physical:** **Behavioral:**
		Emotional: **Physical:** **Behavioral:**

Chapter 6

Session 5: Cognitive Restructuring

Goals

- To review the connection between negative thoughts and pain
- To practice changing negative thoughts into positive coping thoughts

Overview

This session begins with a review of the connection between negative thoughts and pain. In particular, you will look at your pain-specific thoughts and how they affect your experience of pain. You will then learn the process of cognitive restructuring in order to change negative thoughts into more positive ones.

Negative Thoughts and Pain

As discussed in previous chapters, negative thoughts can open the gate to pain. Even though negative thoughts in general are related to increased pain, negative thoughts specifically about pain can have an even greater impact on your experience of pain. Pain-specific thoughts like the following can affect your expectations of your ability to cope with pain:

- *I can't cope with this.*
- *My pain is going to kill me.*
- *This pain is too much for me.*
- *I can't do a thing because of my pain.*
- *My pain is getting the better of me.*
- *I can't do anything right.*

These kind of thoughts can lead to negative feelings (frustration, hopelessness, etc.), which can increase your pain. You can use the ABC model to record the emotional, physical, and behavioral consequences of pain-specific thoughts. Remember, it is the thoughts about an event, either positive or negative, that determine the kinds of emotions you experience. To avoid unnecessary distress and pain, you can learn to identify and change negative thoughts in favor of more positive thoughts.

Restructuring Thoughts

Cognitive restructuring is a method that can be used to change negative emotions, along with the physical and behavioral consequences. It involves recognizing the inaccurate negative thoughts that give rise to negative emotions and substituting more positive coping thoughts.

Follow the steps described here, using the Restructuring Thoughts Worksheet (see figs. 6.1 and 6.2 for completed examples). A blank copy of the worksheet is also provided. You may photocopy this form from the book or download multiple copies from the Treatments-ThatWork™ Web site at www.oup.com/us/ttw. You can use negative thoughts from your previous ABC worksheets for practice.

Steps to Cognitive Restructuring

1. Think of a recent stressful situation that resulted in negative emotions and record this in the first column.

2. Describe and record the emotions you were having at the time (e.g., anxious, frustrated, angry, sad, depressed) and rate the emotion from 0% to 100%.

3. Write down the thoughts (beliefs) you were having that led to the emotions.

4. Pay attention to the description of thoughts. While some of your thoughts may be specifically related to the situation described, others may be more general automatic thoughts based on cognitive errors (e.g., "I never do anything right," "My life is miserable").

5. Evaluate the thoughts.

   ◾ Look for any evidence (facts) that the thought is true.
   ◾ Identify any evidence (facts) that the thought might not be true.

6. If there is evidence to suggest that the thought might not be entirely true, write down a positive coping thought that is more consistent with the facts and evidence (e.g., "I'm learning some great skills to help me take control of my pain," "I don't have to let pain keep me from enjoying myself").

7. Think about the feelings you have when repeating the original negative thought compared to the positive coping thought. If you had been thinking the positive coping thought in that situation, what feelings might have you had instead? How would repeating the positive coping thought affect your physical reactions and behaviors? Rate the emotion from 0% to 100%.

Homework

✎ Practice cognitive restructuring for three thoughts during the week using the Restructuring Thoughts Worksheet. One of the thoughts must be specific to pain.

✎ Work toward completing the weekly behavioral goals set at the end of the session.

Behavioral Goals for the Week

1. _____

2. _____

3. _____

4. _____

5. _____

Situation	Emotion	Automatic Thought	Evidence for	Evidence against	Positive Coping Thought	Emotion
Describe the event that led to the unpleasant emotion.	Specify sad, angry, etc., and rate the emotion from 0% to 100%.	Write the automatic thought that preceded the emotion.	What is the evidence that this thought is true?	What is the evidence that this thought is false?	What else can I say to myself instead of the automatic thought?	Re-rate the emotion from 0% to 100%.
A pain flare-up on a busy day.	Depressed 60% Frustrated 50%	I can't cope with my pain; my life is miserable.	There is too much going on today. I feel overwhelmed and I'm not getting my work done.	I have had busy days before when I've been in pain and I was able to handle my pain and all my responsibilities well. I'm usually very productive. My life isn't all bad (I have a great family).	Not every day is this hectic and some days are good. I have made it through very hectic days before and I can do it again.	Depressed 25% Frustrated 30%

Note that while one of the thoughts is pain-specific, the patient has also brought in an automatic thought about life in general being miserable. With this cognitive error, he discounts the positive aspects of his life.

Figure 6.1

Example of Completed Restructuring Thoughts Worksheet for a Pain-Specific Situation

Situation	Emotion	Automatic Thought	Evidence for	Evidence against	Positive Coping Thought	Emotion
Describe the event that led to the unpleasant emotion.	Specify sad, angry, etc., and rate the emotion from 0% to 100%.	Write the automatic thought that preceded the emotion.	What is the evidence that this thought is true?	What is the evidence that this thought is false?	What else can I say to myself instead of the automatic thought?	Re-rate the emotion from 0% to 100%.
Stuck in line at the grocery store behind someone who is moving slowly.	Angry 50% Frustrated 70%	This always happens to me; I'm going to be here forever. People are so inconsiderate.	I was stuck behind a slow person last time I was here.	There have been times that I've gone through this line very quickly. I know I will not be here forever. The person is probably not doing it on purpose.	A 5-minute delay is not worth getting upset. I can kill a few minutes by reading the magazine covers; I would waste this much time at home anyway.	Angry 20% Frustrated 25%

Note that in this example the person has brought in an automatic thought about people in general being inconsiderate. This cognitive error serves to increase the intensity of the emotions in this situation.

Figure 6.2

Example of Completed Restructuring Thoughts Worksheet for a General Stressful Situation

Restructuring Thoughts Worksheet

Situation	Emotion	Automatic Thought	Evidence for	Evidence against	Positive Coping Thought	Emotion
Describe the event that led to the unpleasant emotion.	Specify sad, angry, etc., and rate the emotion from 0% to 100%.	Write the automatic thought that preceded the emotion.	What is the evidence that this thought is true?	What is the evidence that this thought is false?	What else can I say to myself instead of the automatic thought?	Re-rate the emotion from 0% to 100%.

Chapter 7

Session 6: Stress Management

Goals

- To define stress
- To understand the "fight-or-flight" response
- To identify sources of stress
- To examine the relationship between stress and pain
- To learn ways to decrease stress

Overview

This session describes what stress is and how it affects us. You will learn about the changes that happen in your body as part of the "fight-or-flight" response. By reviewing common sources of stress, you will begin to identify your personal stressors. Last, you will try making changes in your life in order to reduce stress.

What is Stress?

You may think that "stress" is always a bad thing, but it can also be the result of positive events in our lives (e.g., the birth of a child, a new relationship). Any event that requires us to make changes and put forth effort involves a certain amount of stress. Some events, such as deadlines and competitions, may produce feelings of eagerness and excitement, particularly when we think that we have a chance of succeeding. The arousal you feel when you try to meet these challenges is considered healthy.

However, when you perceive a situation or event as being overwhelming, beyond your abilities to cope, and threatening to your well-being, then it is considered "stressful." Stress can result in feelings of exhaustion, fatigue, and depression, which in turn can lead to

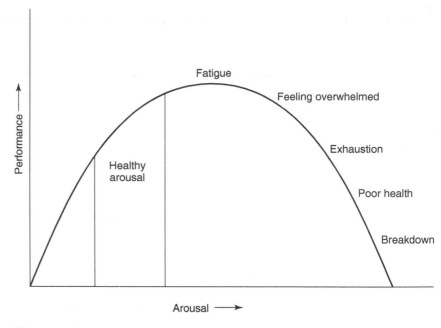

Figure 7.1

Arousal and Performance

health problems such as headaches, upset stomach, and high blood pressure. Stress can also affect work performance and relationships.

The relationship between arousal stress and performance is shown in Figure 7.1. Stress helps us perform, but if we experience too much stress, we begin to break down. Note that it is not the events themselves that cause stress, but how a person reacts to them. In the same situation, one person may feel a healthy amount of arousal, while another person may feel "stressed out."

The Fight-or-Flight Response

Stress is related to a primitive system in our body called the "fight-or-flight" response. It is called this because it provides the strength and energy to either fight or run away from danger. The physical changes that occur when this system is activated include the following:

- An increase in heart rate and blood pressure (to get more blood to the muscles, brain, and heart)

- Faster breathing (to take in more oxygen)

- Tensing of muscles (to prepare for actions like running)

- Increased mental alertness and sensitivity of sense organs (to assess the situation and act quickly)

- Increased blood flow to the brain, heart, and muscles (the organs that are most important in dealing with danger)

- Less blood to the skin, digestive tract, kidneys, and liver (where it is least needed in times of crisis)

- An increase in blood sugar, fats, and cholesterol (for extra energy)

- A rise in platelets and blood clotting factors (to prevent hemorrhage in case of injury)

Although this system was adaptive in the past (e.g., to help our ancestors in hunting), it is not always appropriate today. In fact, when this system is turned on for long periods of time it can have harmful effects on the body (e.g., decreased immune function, heart disease).

Common Sources of Stress

The physical effects of stress are the same for us as they were for our ancestors, but the sources of stress may be different. See Table 7.1 and Table 7.2 for potential external and internal stressors. Note which ones may be a source of stress for you.

Table 7.1 External Stressors

Type	Examples	My Stressors
Physical environment	Noise, bright lights, heat, confined spaces	
Social	Rudeness, bossiness, or aggressiveness on the part of someone else	
Organizational	Rules, regulations, "red tape," deadlines	
Major life events	Death of a relative, lost job, promotion, new baby	
Daily hassles	Commuting, misplacing keys, mechanical breakdowns	

Table 7.2 Internal Stressors

Type	Examples	My Stressors
Lifestyle choices	Caffeine, lack of sleep, overloaded schedule, unhealthy diet	
Negative self-talk	Pessimistic thinking, self-criticism, over-analyzing	
Mind traps	Unrealistic expectations, taking things personally, all-or-nothing thinking, exaggerating, rigid thinking	
Stressful personality traits	Perfectionist, workaholic, have to please others	

Stress and Pain

Stress and pain reinforce each other. You may have noticed that when you are stressed out, your pain gets worse. On the other hand, chronic pain is often a source of stress. This can result in a cycle of pain and stress.

Pain Leads to Stress

Based on the definition of stress discussed earlier in this chapter, a situation is considered stressful only if a person believes that the demands exceed her ability to cope with them. If a person feels that she can handle the sensations of pain and even all of the experiences associated with chronic pain (e.g., disability, job loss, marital problems), she may avoid pain-related stress. However, for many people with chronic pain, it is considered to be a significant source of stress in their lives.

Stress Leads to Pain

Stress is associated with perceptions of limited ability to cope and poor problem-solving skills. These factors can contribute to depression and negative moods, which can increase pain. These may also result in decreased efforts to take personal responsibility for the management of pain. Such a person may be more prone to rely on others (e.g., physicians) to prescribe pain medication or perform some type of intervention to relieve their pain. Feeling a lack of control over pain can raise stress levels, which in turn can lead to increased pain.

Ways to Decrease Stress

Given the relationship between stress and pain, it is important to learn how to manage stress. The good news is that there are things you can do to decrease your stress. This section lists several different kinds of changes you can make. Review these lists and note which ones you want to try on the My Life Changes form.

Change Lifestyle Habits

- Decrease caffeine intake (coffee, tea, colas, chocolate)

- Maintain a balanced diet and decrease consumption of junk food

- Eat slowly and at regular intervals

- Exercise regularly (at least 30 minutes three times per week)

- Get adequate sleep (figure out how much you need)

- Take time-outs and leisure time (do something for yourself every day)

- Do relaxation exercises (e.g., breathing, imagery, PMR)

Change How You Approach Situations

- Time and money management

- Assertiveness (see Chapter 10)

- Problem-solving coping skills

Change your Thinking

- Have realistic expectations (when expectations are more realistic, life seems more manageable)

■ Keep a sense of humor (being able to see the humor in the things helps to lighten the situation)

■ Have a support system (speak with someone or write down your thoughts)

■ Focus on the positive (think half-full versus half-empty)

■ Challenge negative thinking using cognitive restructuring skills (see Chapter 6)

Homework

✎ Identify external and internal stressors in your life. Record these under the "My Stressors" column in Table 7.1 and Table 7.2.

✎ Select changes you would like to try in order to decrease stress. Record these on the My Life Changes form.

✎ Work toward completing the weekly behavioral goals set at the end of the session.

Behaviorial Goals for the Week
1. _____
2. _____
3. _____
4. _____
5. _____

My Life Changes

In the spaces provided, indicate the types of changes you would like to make in your life in order to help decrease stress. Be as specific as possible.

Lifestyle Habits

Diet: _____

Exercise: _____

Sleep: _____

Relaxation: _____

Approaches to Situations

Time management: _____

Money management: _____

Assertiveness: _____

Problem-solving coping skills: _____

Ways of thinking

Realistic expectations: _____

Sense of humor: _____

Support system: _____

Positive thinking: _____

Challenge negative thinking: _____

Other Changes

_____

_____

_____

_____

_____

_____

Chapter 8

Session 7: Time-Based Pacing

Goals

- To learn about time-based pacing
- To practice pacing activities
- To review pacing techniques

Overview

This session introduces a method of pacing activities based on time intervals. You will learn how to estimate how often you need to take breaks in order to effectively manage pain. You will begin to pace some of your activities using the Activity Pacing Worksheet.

Time-Based Pacing

You may find that when you begin a project it is very hard for you to stop working on it before it's completed. You work on the project non-stop despite the onset of pain. As a result of "working through" the pain, the level of your pain becomes higher and higher. This may sometimes result in severe pain that requires you to rest for an extended period, even days, before you are able to work again. Once the pain decreases, you may then feel you have to work extra hard in order to catch up on time lost. You do everything on your "to do" list on that day, only to end up in more pain for days afterwards.

If this sounds familiar, you are not alone. The cycle of work, pain, and rest is very common for individuals who have chronic pain (Fig. 8.1).

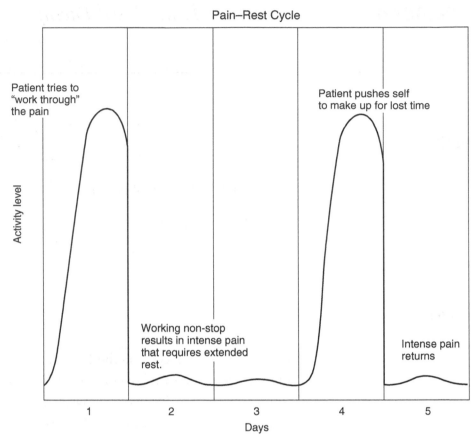

Figure 8.1

Pain-Rest Cycle Graph

One method for breaking this cycle is called *time-based pacing*. Time-based pacing is a process in which activity breaks are based on time intervals, not on how much of the job is completed (Fig. 8.2).

Some people are reluctant to pace themselves because they think they can't afford to "slow down." Actually, though, by taking breaks before pain begins (not after pain gets bad), you will be able to return to activity sooner and will actually get more done. By using time rather than pain as an indicator, you will not need long periods of rest to recover from pain because the pain flare-up will never happen. Professional athletes use pacing by taking regular water breaks on the sidelines in order to perform at peak efficiency. Their coaches know that if players are kept in the game until they are tired, then they will not be performing at their best. The same reasoning applies to you.

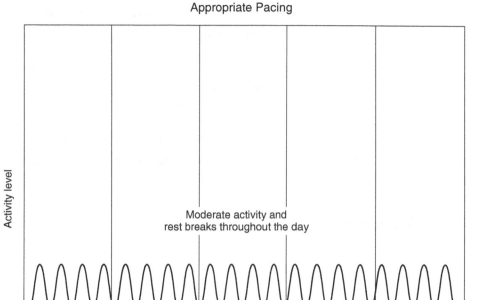

Figure 8.2

Time-Based Pacing Graph

Steps to Time-Based Pacing

Using the Activity Pacing Worksheet, try pacing a few activities in the coming week. You may photocopy this form from the book or download multiple copies from the Treatments *That Work*™ Web site at www.oup.com/us/ttw. Follow these steps:

1. Identify a task that you typically do every day that increases your pain. Or think of something you are planning to do this week that you fear may cause increased pain.

2. Estimate how long you can do the task safely without creating a pain flare-up; this will be your goal "active" time. The

amount of time should be a few minutes less than the point when pain begins.

3. Estimate how long you will need to rest before becoming active again in order to avoid pain flare-ups; this will be called your goal "rest" time.

4. As you perform the activity, record your actual "active" and "rest" times for each day on the Activity Pacing Worksheet on page 58.

Pacing Techniques

When practicing pacing, keep the following in mind:

- Different types of activities require different activity/rest schedules.

- Estimates are not always accurate the first time. Adjust the schedule as you go.

- If flare-ups do occur, cut the activity level in half at first and over three days build back up to the previous level of activity.

- Do not stop practicing time-based pacing skills even when you feel good or pain-free.

Pacing needs to be consistent in order to be an effective pain-reducing strategy.

As you get better at pacing, try expanding the activity/rest schedule to other activities in your day and slowly build up the active time. You may want to incorporate mini-sessions of progressive muscle relaxation, deep breathing, or visual imagery into planned rest periods at work or at home. Other general pacing techniques include:

- Maintain an awareness of your activities and how you do them.

- Avoid rushing and crowded schedules of activities.

- Plan: make a weekly calendar and spread activities evenly throughout the week.

- Make a flexible daily schedule.

- Prioritize activities.

- Set reasonable goals for total activity.

- Use time-contingent rather than pain-contingent termination of activities.

- Use relaxation and other pain coping strategies.

Homework

✎ Practice time-based pacing for several activities using the Activity Pacing Worksheet.

✎ Work toward completing the weekly behavioral goals set at the end of the session.

Behavioral Goals for the Week

1. _____

2. _____

3. _____

4. _____

5. _____

Activity Pacing Worksheet

Activity	GOAL	Day 1	Day 2	Day 3	Day 4	Day 5	Day 6	Day 7
Walking	Active: 7 minutes Resting: 10 minutes	Active: 4 minutes Resting: 15 minutes	Active: 5 minutes Resting: 15 minutes	Active: 9 minutes Resting: 12 minutes	Active: 5 minutes Resting: 12 minutes	Active: 6 minutes Resting: 12 minutes	Active: 7 minutes Resting: 12 minutes	Active: 7 minutes Resting: 10 minutes
	Active: Resting:	Active: Resting:	Active: Resting:	Active: Resting:	Active: Resting:	Active: Resting:	Active: Resting:	Active: Resting:
	Active: Resting:	Active: Resting:	Active: Resting:	Active: Resting:	Active: Resting:	Active: Resting:	Active: Resting:	Active: Resting:
	Active: Resting:	Active: Resting:	Active: Resting:	Active: Resting:	Active: Resting:	Active: Resting:	Active: Resting:	Active: Resting:

Chapter 9

Session 8: Pleasant Activity Scheduling

Goals

- To identify activities that you enjoy

- To schedule pleasant activities

Overview

This session focuses on scheduling pleasant activities. You will choose and plan activities you would like to do. This will help increase your activity level and may reduce negative thoughts and pain.

Pleasant Activity Scheduling

The experience of chronic pain can cause you to withdraw socially or reduce your activity level. Depending on your pain condition, there may be some activities that you can no longer perform like you once could, but you may also have stopped performing some activities for fear of causing more pain. Alternatively, you may avoid some activities or social events because you do not want to answer annoying questions about your pain (e.g., "You don't look like you're in pain; what's wrong with you?"), or because you feel embarrassed or frustrated over your physical limitations. As a result, you may isolate yourself and stop doing the things that you once found the most enjoyable. Without engaging in enjoyable activities and social situations in your life, you are likely to feel depressed, which can further contribute to disability and the experience of pain.

One way to help prevent this from happening is to plan an increased number of pleasant activities throughout the week. The introduction of more positive activities into your routine may help to reduce negative thoughts and emotions, increase overall activity levels, and decrease pain.

The first step is to identify things that you would like to start doing. The second step is to schedule these activities into the week.

Choosing Pleasant Activities

To start, think of activities that you enjoy. This may be more difficult than anticipated, particularly if you have had pain for a long time and are not in the habit of doing enjoyable things for yourself. Its important to remember that there may be things you would *like* to do but are not *able* to do because of physical limitations associated with pain or aging. Though you may not be able to perform the same activities that you could when you were younger, there are often alternative ways of being involved in activities. For example, you may not be able to play 18 holes of golf, but you can probably putt on the putting green; you may not be able to make a three-course meal, but can teach someone else to cook.

Focus on setting achievable and realistic activity goals. The activities can be things that you have done in the recent past and would like to do again, things you have not done for some time, things you have never done but have always meant to do, or activities you would like to perform on a more frequent basis. The Pleasant Activities List can help you come up with ideas.

Pleasant Activities List

1. Having a hobby
2. Relaxing
3. Exercising
4. Reading
5. Sightseeing
6. Listening to music
7. Spending time with friends
8. Playing or watching sports
9. Cleaning
10. Going on a date
11. Traveling
12. Cooking

13. Thinking positive thoughts
14. Dancing
15. Enjoying nature
16. Playing games
17. Eating
18. Repairing things
19. Having family gatherings
20. Writing
21. Playing music
22. Going to a play or lecture
23. Learning something new
24. Taking care of yourself
25. Shopping
26. Telling jokes
27. Playing with animals
28. Taking a class
29. Pampering yourself
30. Going to a museum
31. Talking on the phone
32. Entertaining

33. Collecting things
34. Going for a walk
35. Thinking about good memories
36. Watching children play
37. Singing
38. Organizing
39. Going to a party or event
40. Planning for the future
41. Joining a club
42. Dressing up
43. Daydreaming
44. Taking or looking at pictures
45. Doing arts and crafts
46. Teaching
47. Solving a problem, puzzle, or crossword
48. Volunteering
49. Practicing religion
50. Having a discussion

Scheduling Pleasant Activities

Even though the activity is something fun, you may find yourself procrastinating or avoiding getting started. Make a commitment to doing the activity and schedule it into your week. You may also need to make preparations in order to do the activity. For example, if reading a new book is one of your chosen pleasant activities, you will need to decide what to read, when to read, and get the book ahead of time. Use the Pleasant Activity Schedule worksheet provided to keep track of when you complete your chosen activities. You may photocopy this form from the workbook or download multiple copies from the Treatments *That Work*™ Web site at www.oup.com/us/ttw.

Homework

✎ Schedule at least two pleasant activities for the week using the Pleasant Activity Schedule worksheet.

✎ Work toward completing the weekly behavioral goals set at the end of the session.

Behavioral Goals for the Week
1. _____
2. _____
3. _____
4. _____
5. _____

Pleasant Activity Schedule

1. Choose several pleasant activities that can be scheduled over the course of a week.

2. Place an "X" on each day on which the activity was accomplished.

Paced? Yes/No	Activity	Sunday	Monday	Tuesday	Wednesday	Thursday	Friday	Saturday
Yes	Gardening		X		X		X	

Chapter 10 | *Session 9: Anger Management*

Goals

- To define anger
- To understand the relationship between anger and pain
- To learn how to manage anger

Overview

In earlier sessions, you have learned that negative emotions can have an impact on pain. This session focuses on anger and its relationship to pain. You will learn steps to manage your anger and how to respond to situations more assertively.

What Is Anger?

Anger is a natural emotional response that we all have from time to time. It is an emotion that can range from mild irritation to intense rage. Anger can produce physical changes in the body such as increased heart rate and blood pressure and the release of adrenaline (recall the "fight-or-flight" response discussed in Chapter 7). We can actually feel some of these changes, like tense muscles and a flushed face, as they occur. Anger can also affect our behavior: we might yell, threaten, or attack. The experience of anger is related to the way we think about something that happens. When we are feeling threatened, anger is an adaptive response because it prepares us to attack or defend ourselves.

So if anger is a natural reaction, why do we want to control it? When anger is allowed to go unchecked, it can actually begin to fuel itself and cause more anger. It's hard to think clearly when angry, and you

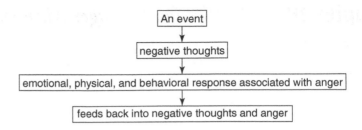

Figure 10.1

Anger Chain Reaction

may say and do things you normally wouldn't, which can lead to regret once your anger has subsided and calmer thoughts are in control. In addition, anger that continues over time can be a source of stress and have a negative impact on the body, including the experience of pain. Figure 10.1 illustrates the chain reaction of anger.

Anger and Pain

You may have noticed that your pain seems worse when you get really angry. There may be several reasons for this. First, anger is often associated with increased muscle tension, which may cause an increase in pain, particularly if the muscle tension is in an area affected by pain. Second, when you experience negative thoughts and emotions related to one situation, it may lead you to focus on all things negative in your life, including pain and its associated problems. If you think of this in terms of the gate control theory discussed earlier, anger may result in an opening of the pain gate, allowing more information about pain to reach the brain. You may have also noticed that when you are in pain, you get mad more easily. Pain lowers the anger threshold for some people, so that even minor irritations set off feelings of anger.

Anger Management

It is important to learn how to keep anger under control. There are three steps to anger management: develop awareness, modify internal responses, and respond assertively.

Step 1: Develop Awareness

Environmental Awareness

Be aware of triggers for anger in your environment, including:

- Verbal/physical abuse or sarcasm (e.g., is there a person who knows just what to say to make you angry?)

- Annoyances and irritations (e.g., excessive noise, interruptions, or minor accidents)

- Common frustrations (e.g., you are prevented, blocked, or disappointed)

- Perceived injustices (e.g., you feel you have been treated unfairly)

Physical Awareness

Be aware of physical changes in your body that can serve as warning signs that you are becoming angry, such as heart racing, muscle tension, making a fist, jaw clenching, or face turning red or warm.

Behavioral Awareness

Be aware of behavior changes, such as pacing back and forth or stiff posture. How we behave when we get angry can determine whether anger will fade or continue to get worse.

Step 2: Modify Internal Responses

Physical

Use relaxation skills like diaphragmatic breathing, progressive muscle relaxation, or imagery when you feel yourself becoming angry. These techniques are helpful to counter the physical changes (e.g., increased heart rate, tense muscles) that occur when you become angry. Try all of these techniques and use the one that works best for you.

Cognitive

▪ Try to consider the feelings of others. Anger often occurs because we assume that we know what other people are thinking and feeling. In reality, we do not; no one can read minds or predict the future.

▪ Think about your own feelings: are you really angry about this, or is it something else?

▪ Use humor to take the edge off anger or to defuse the situation.

▪ Use cognitive restructuring techniques:

1. Identify the automatic thoughts behind the feelings of anger (e.g., "she did that on purpose," "he has always hated me," or "she doesn't care about me").

2. Avoid traps that increase your anger (e.g., believing that everyone is out to get you, thinking that you must have everything your way, exaggerating the importance of an event). This is important because internal conversations can fuel anger and prolong it long after the incident has occurred.

3. Challenge cognitive errors/negative thoughts and generate alternative interpretations of events.

4. Replace unhelpful negative thoughts with more positive coping thoughts.

Step 3: Respond Assertively

The next step is to learn constructive ways that you can take action or express an opinion when you become angry. There are two common response styles that you may use that are not helpful.

Less Adaptive Response Styles

Withdrawal and Avoidance

Do you avoid dealing with conflict or angry emotions? If so, the issue that caused your anger may go unresolved and the negative emotions may be left ready to resurface at another time. Avoidance can even cause your anger to grow and create resentment towards others, as you may continue to think about the event after it has passed. For example, you may think, "What he said was really awful. I shouldn't have let him get away with that."

Aggression, Antagonism, and Hostility

Do you become aggressive or threatening when angry? This type of response can lead others to feel guarded or edgy. The other person may also become hostile if he feels he is being attacked. You may find that you do not get pushed around very often, but no one will want to be around you.

Assertive Responding

This is the best way of responding when you are feeling angry. Assertive behavior means standing up for your rights and expressing what you believe, feel, and want in a direct, honest, and appropriate way that respects the rights of others. The advantage of being assertive is that you can often get what you want, usually without making others angry. If you are assertive, you can act in your own best interest and not feel guilty or wrong about it. An assertive person can express his likes and interests spontaneously, can talk about himself without being self-conscious, can accept compliments comfortably, can disagree with someone openly, can ask for clarification, and can say "no." In short, when you are an assertive person, you can be more relaxed in interpersonal situations.

How to Respond Assertively

- Confront the person you are angry with at an appropriate time and place. Wait until your emotions are under control so that you can communicate more effectively.

- Communicate a willingness to understand the other person's point of view. It's important to be respectful of other people's opinions.

- Using "I" statements, be direct and tell the person why you are angry and what exactly led to your becoming angry. Example of an "I" statement: "I feel angry when you spend a lot of money without talking to me about it first."

Being assertive is not always easy, but it is important for effective communication with others and can help to reduce tension and anger.

Guidelines for Communicating with Others Assertively

1. Maintain eye contact and position your body squarely toward others. Look the other person in the eye most of the time, but do not stare fixedly. Lean forward and use hand gestures to maintain his attention.

2. Speak firmly and positively, and loudly enough to be heard easily. Avoid mumbling, whining, speaking shrilly, or yelling. Avoid dropping your voice at the end of a sentence.

3. Use clear, concise speech. Ask directly for what you want or say clearly what you don't want. Avoid numerous repetitions and qualifiers such as "maybe" or "I guess." Avoid undoing statements such as "I shouldn't ask, but . . ."

4. Make sure your nonverbal behavior matches the content of your statement. Don't smile when refusing or disagreeing. Don't wring your hands when requesting. Avoid a rigid face when expressing warmth or praise.

5. Listen. Repeat the point that the other person made, clarify, or say something that shows that you are listening.

6. Maintain a posture and attitude of equality. Avoid apologetic statements or a tone that belittles yourself or your ideas. Avoid accusing statements or a tone of sarcasm or ridicule. Be respectful of yourself and others.

7. Take the initiative. Don't let others choose for you. Take the lead with, "I have a suggestion . . ." or "In my opinion . . ."

✎ Complete the Restructuring Thoughts Worksheet on page 72 for events that led to feelings of anger.

✎ Work toward completing the weekly behavioral goals set at the end of the session.

Behavioral Goals for the Week
1. _____
2. _____
3. _____
4. _____
5. _____

Restructuring Thoughts Worksheet

Situation	Emotion	Automatic Thought	Evidence for	Evidence against	Positive Coping Thought	Emotion
Describe the event that led to the unpleasant emotion.	Specify sad, angry, etc., and rate the emotion from 0% to 100%.	Write the automatic thought that preceded the emotion.	What is the evidence that this thought is true?	What is the evidence that this thought is false?	What else can I say to myself instead of the automatic thought?	Re-rate the emotion from 0% to 100%.

Chapter 11

Session 10: Sleep Hygiene

Goals

- ▨ To understand the necessity of sleep
- ▨ To learn ways to improve sleep

Overview

Although there are many types of sleep problems that a person may have, common problems for people who have pain include difficulty falling asleep and problems staying asleep due to pain. Even if sleep has not been an issue for you, you can still benefit from a review of good sleep habits. In this session, you will learn why a good night's sleep is necessary and ways to improve your sleep.

Necessity of Sleep

Sleep is an opportunity for our bodies to repair themselves, both physically (e.g., torn muscles, organ cleansing) and psychologically (e.g., working through anxiety). Each sleep cycle (which lasts about 100 minutes) is divided up into physically repairing sleep and psychologically repairing sleep. When we first fall asleep, more time is spent in physically repairing sleep; later in the sleep cycle more time is spent in psychologically repairing sleep. Age influences the balance between these two types of sleep. Babies spend more time in psychologically repairing sleep (dream state) because their bodies don't need much physical repair. Older adults spend more time in physically repairing sleep because their bodies are more vulnerable to damage.

Anxiety, depression, and poor sleep habits can interfere with sleep patterns and disrupt the natural ability of the body to repair itself. If sleep is disrupted for an extended period of time, needed physiological repair cannot take place, which can lead to increased fatigue and pain. Other effects of not getting a good night's sleep include:

- Increased emotional distress and irritability

- Increased clumsiness and poor coordination

- Decreased work performance and memory lapses

- Increased risk of automobile accidents

- Difficulty concentrating

Ways to Improve Sleep

There are many ways you can improve sleep. While there are a number of sleep medications available on the market today, almost all of them have significant side effects and none is meant to be used as a long-term solution to sleep problems. Fortunately, you can often improve your sleep simply by changing some of your nighttime routines. These strategies fall under several categories; try using as many of these strategies as you can in order to see what works for you. Use the Sleep Hygiene Worksheet provided to record your good sleeping habits for the week.

Timing

- Establish a pattern to your sleep by going to bed at the same time each evening and getting out of bed at the same time every day, even on weekends, regardless of how much you have slept.

- Avoid taking naps, but if you do nap make it no more than about 25 minutes. If you have problems falling asleep at night, then you should not take naps.

Sleep Behavior

- Establish a pre-sleep ritual to give your body cues that it is time to slow down (e.g., taking a bath or reading for a few minutes before bed).

- Use the bed only for sleep or for sex (do not use your bed as a desk; do not read, eat, or watch TV in bed).

- If you are unable to sleep for more than 15 minutes, then get out of bed. Lying in bed and feeling frustrated will not help. Engage in a quiet, nonstimulating activity and return to bed when you are sleepy.

- Restrict the amount of time you spend in bed to your usual amount of sleep (e.g., 7 hours) even if you have not slept as well as you would have liked.

Environment Tips

- Sleeping is associated with a decline in core body temperature from a state of relative warmth. You can raise your body temperature by taking a warm bath 20 minutes before bed.

- Fluctuations in room temperature disrupt the dream state, so maintain a steady temperature in the room throughout the night. A cool room is more conducive to sleep than a warm room.

- Eliminate illuminated wall clocks or other sources of light (except perhaps a night light if needed).

Ingestion

- Avoid caffeine (a stimulant) four to six hours before bedtime.

- Avoid nicotine (a stimulant) near bedtime and when waking at night.

- Beware of alcohol use. Though alcohol (a depressant) may initially promote sleep onset, it causes awakenings later in the night.

- If hungry before bed, have a light snack, which may be sleep-inducing. A heavy meal too close to bedtime, however, might interfere with sleep.

Mental Control

■ Avoid mentally stimulating activity just before going to bed (e.g., action movies, stimulating conversation, loud music).

■ Try relaxation techniques such as deep breathing and visual imagery. Relaxation can help you get to sleep.

■ Do mentally quiet tasks such as listening to relaxing music, thinking calming thoughts, and so forth. These can help you get to sleep.

Homework

✎ Use the Sleep Hygiene Worksheet to log sleep habits and strategies over the next week.

✎ Identify the assignments that you have found to be the most effective throughout the program.

✎ Work toward completing the weekly behavioral goals set at the end of the session.

Behavioral Goals for the Week
1. _____
2. _____
3. _____
4. _____
5. _____

Sleep Hygiene Worksheet

Record your use of sleep hygiene strategies over a week. Your goal is to use at least one good sleeping habit from any three categories each night. Check the cell of each habit you used.

Sleep Hygiene Category	Good Sleeping Habits	Sun.	Mon.	Tues.	Wed.	Thur.	Fri.	Sat.
Timing	Set a constant bed time							
	Set a constant wake time							
	Do not take naps							
Sleep Behavior	Have a pre-sleep ritual							
	Use the bed only for sleep							
	If unable to sleep for more than 15 minutes, get out of bed							
Environment	Take a warm bath							
	Keep temperature of room constant							
	Keep bedroom dark							
Ingestion	Avoid caffeine, nicotine, and alcohol before bed							
	Eat a light snack before bed							
Mental Control	Avoid stimulating activities; do mentally quiet tasks							
	Use relaxation techniques (breathing, imagery)							

Total number of habits used per night: _____ _____ _____ _____ _____ _____ _____

Chapter 12

Session 11: Relapse Prevention and Flare-Up Planning

Goals

- To plan for pain flare-ups
- To review your progress
- To set future goals

Overview

During the last 10 sessions, you have learned many different skills to help you manage chronic pain. By continuing to practice these skills, you can help prevent relapses of increased pain. Since not all relapses can be avoided, however, this session addresses how to prepare for a pain flare-up. You will learn how to prepare for flare-ups and how to effectively manage them when they do occur. As this is the last session of treatment, you will also review your progress and set future goals.

Relapse Prevention and Flare-Up Planning

It is likely that you will have a "flare-up" or temporary increase of pain at some point in the future. A flare-up may lead to negative automatic thoughts that affect your mood and activity level (Table 12.1). When a flare-up happens, your first inclination may be to take an extra dose of pain medication. There are times when this approach may be appropriate; however, after completing this program you are also armed with a variety of new skills to manage your pain.

Table 12.1 Typical Components of a Pain Flare-Up

Pain Sensation	Automatic Thoughts	Mood Shift	Result
Marked increase or flare-up in pain sensation	*Expectation:* "I thought I learned ways to decrease my pain." *Loss of control:* "I can't deal with this." *Catastrophizing:* "This is unbearable."	Mood becomes negative (e.g., anxiety, depression)	Decrease in activity

How to Manage a Flare-Up

It is important to have a plan for how to handle flare-ups so you do not abandon everything you have learned when one occurs. Flare-up management can be broken into several stages:

Stage 1: Preparation

- Prepare for a pain flare-up before it occurs.

- Become aware of emotional and physical cues that pain is increasing.

- Rehearse positive statements regarding the ability to cope with pain; reject a helpless attitude.

- Stop negative thoughts and redirect attention to positive coping statements.

Stage 2: Confrontation

- Confront the pain flare-up by using the self-management strategies you have learned in this program.

- Switch strategies as necessary (e.g., imagery, diaphragmatic breathing, and cognitive restructuring).

■ Do not magnify the sensations. Negative thoughts only make the pain seem worse.

■ Use positive coping statements in place of negative thoughts (e.g., "I've handled this much pain before, and I can do it again;" "I won't attempt to totally eliminate the pain, I'll just try to keep it manageable").

Not giving way to negative thinking is critical to managing a pain flare-up. By practicing the strategies learned in this program you can learn to identify negative thoughts and deliberately change them (recall the exercises on identifying cognitive errors and restructuring negative thoughts from sessions 4 and 5). You now have the skills to replace the negative thoughts associated with the pain flare-up with positive coping statements and regain control. Here are some examples:

Thought: "Things are going pretty badly. I can't take it anymore."

Alternate thought: "This has happened before and I know I can get through it. I have planned for this. I'll review the strategies I have put together for dealing with a flare-up and do my best to manage my pain."

Thought: "My pain feels terrible. Things are falling apart just when I thought I was doing well. There is nothing I can do to help myself."

Alternate thought: "I have the ability to manage my pain by using some of the skills I learned in the pain program. I might not be able to get rid of the pain completely but I can bring it down a bit. Just take a slow deep breath."

Stage 4: Reflection and Planning

After the flare-up, congratulate yourself for trying the new strategies and reflect on how it went. Pick out the strategies that worked the best for you and create a plan for how to manage the flare-up next time. For example, you might think to yourself:

1. "I feel great about how I handled that pain flare-up. Even though it was about as bad as it gets for me, I didn't let

negative thoughts get the better of me. Using positive coping statements really helped; I'll do that again next time."

2. "This time I let the pain go too far before I used one of my strategies to cope. Next time I'll catch it earlier and try diaphragmatic breathing at the first sign of pain."

3. "I think I'll make a list of everything that seems to work for me so that I can have it with me as a reminder when my pain starts to flare up next time."

Progress Review

Coping Strategies

At this point, you may have a preference for a particular pain management technique (breathing, PMR, imagery, restructuring thoughts, etc.). It's fine to use one strategy more than others, but keep in mind that some skills require time to learn and it is often good to have a variety of skills to choose from.

Treatment Goals

Review the overall treatment goals you set at the beginning of therapy. Were you able to consistently complete the weekly behavioral goals? If not, why? Decide which goals you need to continue working on after the program has ended.

Therapy Termination

Congratulations! You have now completed the pain management program. This, however, does not signal the end of your progress. You will now become your own coach as you continue to work toward your goals. With regular practice, you will improve on the skills you have learned to help you take greater control of your pain.

About the Author

Dr. John D. Otis is an Associate Professor of Psychiatry and Psychology at Boston University. He is the Director of Pain Research and Pain Psychology at the VA Boston Healthcare System, Boston, MA. He received his PhD in Clinical Psychology from the University of Florida, specializing in the assessment and treatment of chronic pain. He currently has several funded research projects, including a research study investigating the efficacy of an intensive CBT treatment for veterans with comorbid chronic pain and posttraumatic stress disorder (PTSD). Dr. Otis has published numerous scholarly articles and book chapters about pain throughout the lifespan, with a focus on the development of innovative approaches to pain management tailored to specialized patient populations.